Mirelys Pazo Rodríguez

Early diagnosis of CKD

Mirelys Pazo Rodríguez

Early diagnosis of CKD

in CMF 19-47 at-risk population.

ScienciaScripts

Imprint

Any brand names and product names mentioned in this book are subject to trademark, brand or patent protection and are trademarks or registered trademarks of their respective holders. The use of brand names, product names, common names, trade names, product descriptions etc. even without a particular marking in this work is in no way to be construed to mean that such names may be regarded as unrestricted in respect of trademark and brand protection legislation and could thus be used by anyone.

Cover image: www.ingimage.com

This book is a translation from the original published under ISBN 978-613-9-40411-7.

Publisher:
Sciencia Scripts
is a trademark of
Dodo Books Indian Ocean Ltd. and OmniScriptum S.R.L publishing group

120 High Road, East Finchley, London, N2 9ED, United Kingdom
Str. Armeneasca 28/1, office 1, Chisinau MD-2012, Republic of Moldova, Europe
Printed at: see last page
ISBN: 978-620-7-69382-5

TITLE: COMMUNITY INTERVENTION FOR THE EARLY DIAGNOSIS OF CHRONIC KIDNEY DISEASE IN THE POPULATION AT RISK OF CMF 19-47.

POLICLÍNICO "CAPITÁN ROBERTO FLEITES"

AUTHORS

Dr. Luis Antonio Caballero Sardiñas Dr. Mirelys Pazo Rodríguez Dr. Mileidy Pazo Rodríguez

Dr. Carmen Moré Chang Dr. Idalmis Elena Vázquez López

Dr. Yamile Álvarez Luna

Lic. María de los Ángeles Madrigal Castro

Faculty of Medicine. University of Medical Sciences of Villa Clara. Cuba.

E-mail: mirelyspr@infomed.sld.cu 15 May 2024

INDEX

AUTHORS 2

INTRODUCTION 6

OBJECTIVES 11

METHODOLOGICAL DESIGN 12

RESULTS 19

DISCUSSION AND RESULTS 26

CONCLUSIONS 33

RECOMMENDATIONS 34

BIBLIOGRAPHICAL REFERENCES 35

ANNEXES 43

SUMMARY

Introduction: Chronic Kidney Disease (CKD) is currently considered a catastrophic disease due to the increase in cases, affects a significant percentage of the population and is related to phenomena or diseases of high prevalence such as Arterial Hypertension and Diabetes Mellitus. Objective: To contribute to the early diagnosis of CKD in the population at risk, belonging to CMF 19-47 of the Policlínico Universitario, Capitán Roberto Fleites. Methodology: A descriptive cross-sectional study was carried out with the aim of contributing to the early diagnosis of CKD in the at-risk population belonging to CMF 19-47 of the University Polyclinic, Captain Roberto Fleites in the period November 2020 to May 2023.Results: A total of 17 patients in early stages of CKD were diagnosed, representing 16.5 % of the patients at risk population studied, of whom 82.3 % were in stage II and 58.8 % were patients with arterial hypertension.Conclusions: A low level of knowledge predominated, a number of patients in the initial stages of CKD were diagnosed in Primary Health Care, through the results of serum creatinine and calculation of Glomerular Filtration, the relationship of Arterial Hypertension and Diabetes Mellitus as the main entities associated with the development of CKD was demonstrated.

Keywords: Chronic kidney disease, early diagnosis, at-risk population, glomerular filtration rate, community intervention

INTRODUCTION

The epidemiological view of Chronic Kidney Disease (CKD) has undergone a notable change in the last twenty years. Initially restricted to entities of relatively low incidence, such as glomerular diseases or hereditary nephropathies, and to a specialised field of care (Nephrology), it now affects a significant percentage of the population and is related to diseases of high prevalence, such as Arterial Hypertension (AHT), Diabetes Mellitus (DM) or Cardiovascular Disease[1, 2].

The first references to kidney pathologies date back to ancient Egypt (1500 BC), but it is Hippocrates of Cos (Greece; 460 - 370 BC) who first recognised and described various subtle macroscopic changes in the urine, which indicate specific diseases in different organs, primarily the kidney. According to Hippocrates, no other system or organ of the human body can give more diagnostic information by inspection than the urinary system with the urine produced by the diseased kidney[3,4].

It is currently considered a catastrophic disease due to the increase in the number of cases, the cost of treating it and the fact that it is diagnosed when it has already developed; it is an increasingly frequent clinical condition that affects around 10% of the world's population according to reports of studies included in the literature reviewed. It is included in the group of non-communicable or emerging diseases, as a result of epidemiological and demographic transitions and its high impact on the population, constituting a major public health problem [5-8].

In recent decades, there has been a change in the epidemiological pattern of the world's population with a predominance of the ageing process and, as a consequence, the contribution to the appearance of renal pathologies.The epidemiological expression of these diseases in the world population is like the vision of the ice floe of which only a small part is visible, the greater proportion remains submerged and its magnitude unknown. It is estimated that for every patient reaching the terminal stage of the disease, there are 200 patients in different stages of the disease, most of them undiagnosed, whose prevalence rate lies at the base of the pyramid; primary health care[9-11].

Epidemic behaviour means that tens of thousands or hundreds of thousands of people and their families are affected in one country. The human costs and the costs of renal replacement therapy transform the individual and family problem into a social and political problem. It has a continuously growing prevalence in most countries of the world, for example in Central America, with a high percentage of the population living with the disease and attending renal replacement therapy on a daily basis. It is one of the diseases that most affects the budget of health ministries and the results are poor. This is why a systemic clinical epidemiological and intersectoral approach is needed for prevention, treatment and rehabilitation [5,10].

It should be considered that the criteria used for the diagnosis of CKD in adults depend on the type of population under study and its magnitude, differentiating the evolutionary stages. In stage V, the predominant aetiology is DM, which reaches frequencies of 50% to 60% in some communities or countries, followed by hypertension (in others, the first), primary and secondary nephropathies (glomerulopathies, congenital, obstructive diseases) and renal transplant failure [12,13].

In Spain, it is estimated that 9.24% of the adult population suffers from some degree of CKD, the percentage of the general population being 6.83% in stages III - V. Its prevalence is increasing due to the ageing of the population, the increase in risk factors such as cardiovascular disease, diabetes mellitus, arterial hypertension or obesity and, obviously, due to its early diagnosis[9]. Studies conducted by several institutions have shown that In the United States, it is estimated that 30 million people, equivalent to 15% of older adults, suffer from this pathology. In Latin America, countries such as Chile and Colombia show prevalence statistics of 5.8% and 2.8% respectively. In Mexico, according to estimated data, there is an incidence of 377 cases per million inhabitants, with an estimated 52,000 patients undergoing renal replacement therapy, 80% of whom are treated at the Mexican Social Security Institute (Instituto Mexicano del Seguro Social). Similarly, Argentina has had for many years a sustained growth in the prevalence of patients on renal replacement therapy. In recent years, this growth has slowed down to around 3%, with a prevalence of 632 patients per million inhabitants and a national incidence of 128 patients per 100,000 inhabitants -[1417] .

This pathology is potentially preventable and its early diagnosis makes it possible to treat the causes and act on the factors of progression in order to delay it, or return to previous stages, favouring the dispensation and follow-up of the patient, the adequate treatment of comorbidities, as well as the prevention and treatment of multisystemic complications.[11] According to warnings from the World Health Organisation (WHO) and the Pan American Health Organisation (PAHO), one in ten people has some degree of CKD, but difficulties persist in terms of its management, such as: late diagnosis, lack of awareness of the disease by health personnel who are not nephrologists, fragmentation of care, late referral, therapeutic nihilism in the progression of the disease and complications, as well as the abrupt start of replacement therapy[17] .

The incidence and prevalence of CKD, caused mainly by the complications of diabetes and hypertension, has increased throughout the Americas, while its morbidity and mortality among the adult population of Latin America has grown in the last 20 years, generating international calls[16-18] .In Cuba, an increase in mortality from glomerular and renal diseases is observed, where in 2017 983 deaths for a rate of 8.7 per hundred thousand people,[19] and in 2019, 1,243 deaths are reported for a rate of 11.1 per hundred thousand people[20] .

The research carried out generally refers to some of the complications of CKD, but the size of the samples and the simultaneous inclusion of incident and prevalent patients make comparisons difficult and limit the potential of this information for epidemiological research, planning and improving the quality of care. Today, Villa Clara is among the provinces with high proportions of patients diagnosed with CKD, and according to a recent study, most cases are diagnosed when the disease has progressed· . Despite having primary care in each community that is responsible for dispensing each patient and thus being able to act appropriately on risk factors, the incidence persists and in general, little can be achieved[21] .

The "Capitán Roberto Fleites" Polyclinic in the Santa Clara municipality, according to the process of dispensation carried out by the basic health teams, in 2019 there were a total of 3497 patients with Diabetes Mellitus, of whom only 18 were diagnosed with CKD; 19,569 with Arterial Hypertension and none with the disease, for a total of 109 people with CKD, with a higher incidence in age groups over 60 years of age. The Family Medical Clinic (CMF) 19-47 also has patients considered to be at high risk of developing the disease. Primary Health Care (PHC) is basically aimed at preventing the emergence of diseases and the prevention of complications in some of them, but this is difficult in CKD due to its multifactorial origin. For this reason, the need for changes in healthy lifestyles should be promoted and disseminated among the high-risk population, through community intervention, aimed at raising awareness of the disease and its timely diagnosis, in order to improve their quality of life and reduce morbidity, which motivated this research aimed at resolving the following scientific problem: How to contribute to the early diagnosis of Chronic Kidney Disease in the population at risk, belonging to CMF 19-47 of the Policlínico Universitario, Capitán Roberto Fleites?

OBJECTIVES

General Objective

- To contribute to the early diagnosis of CKD in the population at risk, belonging to CMF 19-47 of the University Polyclinic, Captain Roberto Fleites.

Specific Objectives

- Characterise patients according to variables of interest in the study.

- To determine the level of information on   CKD in the study group.

- Evaluate renal function studies in at-risk populations for early diagnosis of CKD.

- Assess the community intervention designed by specialist criteria.

METHODOLOGICAL DESIGN

A quasi-experimental study will be carried out with the aim of contributing to the early diagnosis of CKD in the population at risk, belonging to CMF 19-47 of the Policlínico Universitario, Capitán Roberto Fleites in the period November 2020 to May 2023.

Context of the research

The research was conducted in the CMF 19-47 of the Policlínico Universitario, Capitán Roberto Fleites in the period November 2020 to May 2023, the primary data will be collected in the period June 2021 to July 2022.

Population and sample

The study population consisted of 432 patients seen at the CMF, from which the patients at risk who met the research criteria were selected, a total of 103 patients, so the sampling was non-probabilistic and intentional.

Inclusion criteria

Patients over 30 years of age, of both sexes. Who present risk factors for CKD.
Willingness to participate in research, subject to informed consent.

Exclusion criteria

Patients diagnosed with CKD.

Research Methods

In order to solve the scientific problem and achieve the research objectives, the following theoretical and empirical methods were selected:

Theoretical:

- Historical-logical: this was used to analyse the concepts and references related to CKD, which contributed to the formulation of the research problem. In addition, with this method it was possible to learn about the background of research carried out on this subject and how this phenomenon has been handled historically by researchers, making it viable to fulfil the proposed objectives.

- Analysis and synthesis: this was used to evaluate, from different perspectives, the main contributions of foreign and Cuban scholars on CKD, as well as to summarise and integrate the central ideas and generalise the fundamental trends in the understanding of the essential problems currently faced by society in relation to this subject.

- Induction-deduction: was used to guide the entire research process and deduce new conclusions, inferring that the study will make it possible to diagnose CKD in at-risk patients.

Empirical:

- Documentary review was used to analyse the family health records and individual medical history to identify patients with risk factors for CKD.

- Survey: A survey developed by the author of the research was used to identify patients' level of knowledge about CKD.

- Questionnaire to specialists: this was designed so that the designated specialists could provide their assessment of the Community Intervention designed.

Ethical Requirements

In research involving human subjects, it is essential that ethical principles are taken into account and considered by the research professional.

- Principle of Autonomy: Informed Consent was given to the patients in order to obtain their approval and willingness to take part in the research, and they could also withdraw from the research at any time they chose.

- Principle of Beneficence: During the research no act of harm was done to the research participants, attention was paid to their needs, motivations, opinions and reflections, these being the most important for the researcher. They were provided with a space of trust and confidentiality that met the necessary conditions for the optimal development of the study.

- Principle of Justice: Equal opportunities and attention were given to all equally, with no discriminatory actions on any grounds in the investigation.

Investigation Procedure

The research was carried out in four stages. In the first stage, the theoretical and methodological references were reviewed, analysed and defined to address the problem in question, and the research process was also planned, and the population at risk of CKD was identified. This was followed by a research orientation stage, the application of a survey, a semi-structured interview and a physical examination that included indications for complementary tests. In the third stage, the results obtained were analysed and processed. In the fourth stage, the designed community intervention was submitted for assessment by specialists to confirm its feasibility.

Specialists:

- 3 specialists in 1st Degree MGI. Teaching category and 10 years of experience.

- 1 specialist in 1st Degree Nephrology. Teaching category and 10 years of experience.

- 1 graduate in psychology. Teaching category and 10 years of experience.

The variables proposed to achieve the proposed objectives are listed and operationalised below.

- Variable:

Age Group (continuous quantitative) is the time elapsed from birth to the time of entry recorded in revised documents. Measurement: In whole numbers with unit of measurement in years, according to the ranges:

Under 30 years old

30 - 39 years old

40 - 49 years old

50 - 59 years old

60 - 69 years 70 years and over

Indicators: Absolute frequency, relative frequency, extreme values and mean.

- Variable: Sex (qualitative nominal) relates to the biological phenotype observed and recorded in reviewed documents.

Measurement: In the categories:

- Male

- Female

Indicators: Absolute and relative frequency.

- Variable: Skin colour (qualitative nominal) is the characteristics according to skin pigmentation observed and recorded in reviewed documents.

Measurement: In the categories:

White Black Mongrel

Indicators: Absolute and relative frequencies

- Variable: Level of schooling (qualitative nominal) this includes the last expired school grade referred by the patient that completes the level of schooling in which it is included as recorded in documents reviewed.

Measurement: In the categories:

Primary Secondary Secondary Pre-university University

Indicators: Absolute and relative frequencies.

- Variable: Personal pathological history is based on health status.

Measurement: In the categories:

Diabetes Mellitus type 1 Diabetes Mellitus type 2 Arterial Hypertension Nephropathies

Obesity Smoking Dyslipidaemia Urinary tract infection

- Variable: Nutritional assessment (continuous quantitative) is classified according to the body mass index calculated by the expression BMI= weight (kg) [height (m)]^2 ; the values of weight and height recorded in the individual clinical history are required.

Measurement: In the categories:

Underweight: (if BMI < 20.0 kg/m2)

Underweight: (if 20.0 kg/m2 ≤ BMI < 25.0 kg/m2) Overweight: (if 25.0 kg/m2 ≤ BMI < 30.0 kg/m2) Obese: (if BMI ≥ 30.0 kg/m2)

Indicators: Absolute and relative frequency

- Variable: Complementary tests (continuous quantitative) is the value obtained in the complementary tests performed on admission recorded in reviewed documents.

Creatinine. In whole numbers with unit of measurement in µmol/L-.

. Normal value44,2 µmol/L - 132,6 µmol/L

. Stage III132,6 µmol/L - 442 µmol/L

. Stage IV442 µmol/L - 884 µmol/L

. Stage V> 884 µmol/L)

Indicators: Absolute frequency, relative frequency, extreme values and mean.

- Variable: CKD stage (qualitative nominal) is the classification according to the glomerular filtration rate values diagnosed during the investigation. Kidney damage with normal GFR≥ 90 mL/minStage IMild89-60 mL/min Stage II

Moderate59-30 mL/min Stage III

Severe29-15 mL/minStage IV

End-stage renal damage (dialysis)< 15 mL/minStage V

- Variable: Renal Ultrasound Report describes the health condition

Measurement: In categories:

. No Alterations

. Renal Cysts

. Hydronephrosis

. Loss of cortico-medullary relationship

. Polycystic Kidney

. Renal Lithiasis

. Not done

- Variable: Information level is the state of information they possess, according to answers obtained from the questionnaire and semi-structured interview.

Categories:

High:80-100% of correct answers Medium:80- 60% of correct answers Low:< 60% of correct answers

Table 1. Distribution of the sample studied according to age group and sex.
CMF 19-47 Policlínico Capitán Roberto Fleites. January 2021 - May 2023.

Age groups	Sex				Total	
	Female		Male			
	No	%	No	%	No	%
30-39	2	1,9	3	2,9	5	4,8
40-49	5	4,8	11	10,6	16	15,5
50-59	9	8,7	16	15,5	25	24,2
60-69	15	14,5	23	22,3	38	36,8
≥ 70	5	4,8	14	13,5	19	18,4
Total	36	34,9	67	65	103	100

Source: Survey

With regard to age and sex, this is reflected in table 1, where we can see that there was a predominance of the group aged between 60 and 69 years, with 38 cases for 36.8 %, followed by the group aged between 50 and 59 years, which represented 24.2 %. There was a higher representation of the male sex in the study with 67 cases representing 65 per cent.

Table 2. Distribution of the sample studied according to Demographic Variables

CMF 19-47 Policlínico Capitán Roberto Fleites January 2021 - May 2023.

Level of schooling	No	%
Primary	1	0,97
Secondary	35	33,9
Pre-university	40	38,8
University	23	22,3
Illiterate	4	0,88
Total	103	100
Skin colour	No	%
White	88	85,4
Black	9	8,7
Mongrel	5	4,8
Total	103	100

Source: Survey

Table 2 shows the patients according to general characteristics. It could be seen that there was a majority of those with white skin colour with 88 cases representing 85.4 per cent. Those with pre-university education predominated with 40 cases representing 38.8 per cent, followed by those with secondary education with 35 for 33.9 per cent.

Table 3. Distribution of the sample studied according to Personal Pathological History and Sex. CMF 19-47 Policlínico Capitán Roberto Fleites January 2021 - May 2023.

Personal Pathological History	Sex				Total	%
	Female		Male			
	No	%	No	%		
Diabetes Mellitus type 1	1	0,97	0	0	1	0,97
Diabetes Mellitus type 2	7	6,79	14	13,5	21	20,3
Arterial Hypertension	16	15,5	36	34,9	52	50,4
Nephropathies	0	0	1	0,97	1	0,97
Obesity	7	6,79	2	1,94	9	8,73
Smoking	2	1,94	12	11,6	14	13,5
Dyslipidemias	1	0,97	1	0,97	2	1,94
Urinary tract infection	2	1,94	1	0,97	3	2,91
Total	36	34,9	67	65,0	103	100

Source: Survey

Table 3 shows the distribution of patients according to personal pathological history, in which a marked predominance of patients with arterial hypertension was observed (50.4 %), with a higher proportion of male patients (36). This was followed by diabetes mellitus, which accounted for 20.3 %.

Table 4. Distribution of the sample studied according to Personal Pathological History and Sex. CMF 19-47 Policlínico Capitán Roberto Fleites January 2021 - May 2023.

Nutritional Classification	No	%
Normo weight	26	25,2
Overweight	46	44,6
Obese	31	30
Total	103	100

Table 4 shows, according to the calculation of the Body Mass Index, that overweight patients predominate in our risk population, representing 44.6 % of the total, followed by obese patients with a value of 30 %.

Table 5. Distribution of the sample studied according to CKD Stages and Sex. CMF 19-47 Policlínico Capitán Roberto Fleites January 2021 - May 2023.

ERC Stadium	Sex				Total	%
	Female		Male			
	No	%	No	%		
Stage I	1	5,88	2	11,7	3	17,6
Stage II	4	23,5	10	58,8	14	82,3
Total	5	29,4	12	70,5	17	100

Table 5 shows the patients diagnosed in the different stages of CKD, according to the results according to the Cockcroft-Gault equation, with a predominance of patients in Stage II, with 14 patients for 82.3 **%, of whom** 10 are male and only 3 patients are in Stage I of CKD.

Table 6. Distribution of the sample studied according to Personal Pathological History and Chronic Kidney Disease Stages. CMF 19-47 Policlínico Capitán Roberto Fleites January 2021 - May 2023.

Personal Pathological History	ERC Stages		Total	%
	Stage I	Stage II		
Diabetes Mellitus type 2	1	5	6	35,2
Arterial Hypertension	1	9	10	58,8
Nephropathies	1	0	1	5,88
Total	3	14	17	100

Source: Survey

Table 6 shows that 58.8% of patients diagnosed with CKD have hypertension, 9 of them in stage II, followed by 35.2% with type 2 diabetes mellitus, 5 of them diagnosed in stage II.

Table 7. Distribution of the sample studied according to Personal Pathological History and Chronic Kidney Disease Stages. CMF 19-47 Policlínico Capitán Roberto Fleites January 2021 - May 2023.

Age groups	ERC Stages		Total	%
	Stage I	Stage II		
50-59	0	2	2	11,7
60-69	3	6	9	52,9
≥ 70	0	6	6	35,2
Total	3	14	17	100

Table 7 shows that 52.9% of patients diagnosed in the early stages of CKD belong to the 60-69 age group and 35.2% are over 70 years of age.

Table 8. Distribution of the sample studied according to Renal Ultrasound Report and Chronic Kidney Disease Stages. CMF 19-47 Policlínico Capitán Roberto Fleites January 2021 - May 2023.

Renal Ultrasound Report	ERC Stages		Total	%
	Stage I	Stage II		
Quite Renal	1	4	5	29,4
Hydronephrosis	0	2	2	11,7
RCM loss	0	8	8	47
Renal Lithiasis	2	0	2	11,7
Total	3	14	17	100

On the other hand, table 8 shows the results of Renal Ultrasound applied to patients diagnosed with CKD, where we can observe that 47.0 % presented loss of the cortico-medullary relationship and 29.4 % with the presence of renal cysts.

Table 9. Distribution of the sample studied according to Level of Information. CMF 19-47 Policlínico Capitán Roberto Fleites January 2021 - May 2023.

Level Information	No	%
High	5	4,8
Medium	23	22,3
Under	75	72,8
Total	103	100

The application of a survey to our at-risk population showed that 72.8% of the total had a low level of knowledge about CKD, with only 4.8% having a high level of knowledge about the disease. Community intervention for the early diagnosis of chronic kidney disease in the at-risk population of CMF 19-47. Policlínico "Capitán Roberto Fleites".

Activity 1

Identification of patients with chronic non-communicable diseases that may cause CKD, through the family health record and individual history.

Activity 2

Application of a survey and semi-structured interview with patients and physical examination for nutritional assessment. Indication of complementary tests (Creatinine).

Activity 3

Analysis of complementary results and application of the Cockcroft-Gault formula for glomerular filtration rate assessment, which allows identification of CKD and classification according to stage.

Activity 4

Assessment of patients diagnosed by renal ultrasound and evaluation according to sonographic findings.

Activity 5

Discussion with community leaders about the main results of the study, educational talk about CKD and its impact on the community.

Chronic kidney disease is asymptomatic. When the person undergoes a medical examination and complementary diagnostic tests for any ailment, this is when the problem is detected and different health actions should be taken to prevent its progression. This was the motivation and justification for the present study, which included a sample of 103 patients, predominantly male, with a history of arterial hypertension and stage II chronic kidney disease. With regard to the results on the sex of the sample, as shown in table 1, it coincides with a study carried out by Medina[22] , in Nicaragua in 2022, where a marked predominance of the male sex is observed with 83 patients with 54.3%. It does not agree with the study carried out by Panduro Saavedra[23] , in Peru in 2021, where a majority of the female sex was observed with 112, 55% of cases. Moreno and collaborators[24] , in Cuba, in 2020, in their article the female sex with 110 patients with 64.3% showed a greater number, which does not correspond with the present study. They are not similar in a study carried out by Soto Cruzado[25] in 2023, where a predominance of female patients is observed with 122 cases with 62.56%. They do not coincide with a study carried out by Sánchez Castañón[26] in 2023, where a predominance of female patients was observed with 99 cases with 78.6%. The researcher of the present study considers that this result could be related to the fact that many studies show that this disease is more prevalent in the female sex, which is the opposite of what was observed in this research.With regard to the results on the level of schooling of the sample, shown in table 2, they do not agree with a study carried out by Medina[22] , in Nicaragua in 2022, where a marked predominance of the study group with primary schooling was observed, with 90 patients with 58.8%. On the other hand, in an article by Li, W. Y., et al.[27,] in 2020, The majority of the study group with a college or university education is observed with 20 patients with 80%, which does not correspond to the present study.Okoro, et al.[28] , in 2020, obtained a higher number of patients with tertiary school level with 75 patients with 34.1%, which disagrees with the present study. In the present study, it is considered that subjects with a lower level of education are more likely not to understand prevention measures, both sporadically and habitually, compared to those with university studies. The educational level of the population is important to trace the educational actions and to analyse to what extent they can assimilate and change inadequate lifestyles, adopting the total abandonment of unhealthy habits. With regard to the results obtained on the age groups of the sample, as can be seen in table 1, in an article by Okoro and collaborators[28] , in 2020, a predominance of patients aged between 40 and 64 years was observed with 150 cases with 68.2%, which corresponds to the present study. They are similar to a study conducted by Soto Cruzado[25] , in 2023, where a predominance of patients aged between 60 and 65 years is observed with 73 cases with 37.44%. In an article by Moreno, et al.[24] , in Cuba, in 2020, there was a predominance of patients under 50 and between 60 and 69 years of age with 57 patients with 33.3 % respectively, which disagrees with the present study. According to Serra-Valdés et al.[29] , in their article, in 2018, patients over 60 years of age predominated. Medical wards are currently dominated by admissions of patients in the geriatric age group due to the increase in life expectancy in the Cuban population. The systemic ageing process is implicit in age groups over 60 years of age, and this population is generally comorbid; these are ages in which there are chronic non-communicable diseases such as

AHT, DM, and other cardiovascular and cerebrovascular diseases, resulting from the process of atherosclerosis. As for the results on the personal pathological history and sex of the sample, shown in table 3, in an article by Moreno and collaborators[24] , in Cuba, in 2020, a marked predominance of patients with arterial hypertension for 10 or more years was observed, with 60 cases for 85.9%, which disagrees with the present study. Barreto et al.[30] state that 85% of patients with arterial hypertension, after 7 years of evolution, are likely to express renal damage, this being mainly due to structural changes occurring at the level of the juxtaglomerular apparatus, evidenced by glomerular sclerosis.Delgado-Mejía et al.[31] , consider that there is evidence that strict control of blood pressure levels can have a favourable impact by preventing the development of microalbuminuria and thus preventing nephropathy, as well as significantly reducing fatal outcomes due to cardiovascular and cerebrovascular disease. The same study concluded that the findings described above could be used to consider adjusting treatment based on the patient's blood pressure. Classical texts, of course, by authors of other nationalities in whose countries there is a different prevalence of diseases, point out that DM is the most frequent cause of CKD, followed by HTN. However, health statistics in Cuba are different[31] .

In this study, AHT is considered to be the most important modifiable risk factor for developing chronic kidney disease, because it promotes atherosclerosis. Annual screening (by the family doctor) of the diabetic and hypertensive population with low-cost techniques - such as microalbuminuria and creatinine to calculate GFR, dispensing and analysis in the health situation of each community - together with the out-of-hospital extension of nephrology in specialised consultations may contribute to changing this situation.Primary health care (PHC) can contribute to preventing the occurrence of chronic non-communicable disease (NCD) risk factors through health promotion strategies and community participation, or to their prevention. modification; to proactively identify and treat subclinical high-risk patients early through interventions with strategies that have proven to be effective. The high costs of end-stage disease replacement therapy and increased cardiovascular events as a complication, high costs of frequent hospital admissions, premature mortality and reduced quality of life justify the above considerations. With regard to the results shown in table 5 on the stage of chronic kidney disease and sex, they do not coincide with the study carried out by Panduro Saavedra[23] , in Peru in 2021, if we consider the 112 female patients, 54% were in stage III, 37% in stage II and 9% in stage I. In the male group, 55% of the 89 patients were in stage III, 30% in stage II and 9% in stage III. II and 15% in stage I. These results coincide with those of Rodríguez and Herrera[32] , where they indicate that, in Peru, of the 30 patients with renal damage, 36.66% were female, in relation to sex. According to Labrador P, et al.[33] , Primary Care is key in the detection and stratification of CKD, glomerular filtration rate and albuminuria should be used for correct management; even so, the determination of albuminuria is still under-requested, with only 1 in 6 patients seen in Primary Care being correctly stratified. This study demonstrates the importance of being able to diagnose chronic kidney disease at an early stage, which contributes to a better evolution and therefore fewer complications for the patient.On the other hand, the results on personal pathological history and stages of chronic kidney disease in the sample are shown in table 6. According to Kalantar-Zadeh[34] , the main risk factors for developing CKD are diabetes mellitus and arterial hypertension, which is why adequate glycaemic and blood pressure controls must be achieved. Other risk factors for CKD such as obesity, cardiac pathologies, family history of CKD, advanced age and previous kidney damage should also be taken into account[35] .

The important points in this type of prevention are intervention in modifiable factors such as healthy lifestyles: regular physical activity, obesity control, smoking cessation and a diet low in sodium and protein. It is also essential to maintain adequate hydration and to be careful with special conditions such as single-sex patients, adult polycystic disease, etc.[34] .Chen T, et al.[36] , state that, since the initial stages of CKD are asymptomatic, prevention at this stage seeks to detect those who have the disease, for which it is suggested to screen for certain alterations in laboratory tests such as microalbuminuria, haematuria and elevated creatinine and cystatin C levels. This phase is crucial as the AusHEART study showed that only 18% of individuals with impaired renal function were correctly diagnosed with CKD. Interventions in this second phase aim to slow the progression of CKD through two main pillars: reducing the severity of proteinuria and lowering intraglomerular pressure, which is achieved by implementing pharmacological and dietary measures.[34.]

According to Hidalgo Quijije, and collaborator[37] , in a study conducted in Ecuador in 2022, it was observed that the comorbidities associated with renal damage, the most commonly found were diabetes mellitus and hypertension, which can cause damage or injury to the bladder or urethra. In addition to these, there is also smoking, obesity and age, the latter generally being more common in older adults. As for the results on the age groups and stages of CKD in the sample, as shown in table 7. In an article by Domínguez and collaborators[38] , in Matanzas, Cuba in 2021, a greater predominance of patients between 60 and 69 years of age in stage II is observed with 25%. This does not coincide with the study carried out by Panduro Saavedra, N. P.,[23] in Peru in 2021, if we look at the group over 55 years of age, 32% in stage I, 38% in stage II and 29% in stage III a. In an article by Moreno, et al[24], in Cuba, in 2020, a predominance of stages III A and III B was observed from the age of 50 onwards. It should be noted that they found patients in stages III A - III B and stage II under 50 years of age, which does not correspond to the present study. The researcher of the present study points out that as age increases, there is a greater probability that chronic kidney disease will be diagnosed in higher stages, and that more complications will arise. With regard to the results shown in table 8 on sonographic signs and stages of chronic kidney disease in the sample, they do not agree with a study conducted by Vidal Morales[39], in Guatemala in 2020, where it was found that 29% of patients had hydronephrosis, 21% had renal lithiasis, 21% had renal cysts and 3% had polycystic kidneys. From the findings of the article by Raju, et al[40], in India, in 2019, it was concluded that there is a decrease in longitudinal size, parenchymal thickness and cortical thickness along with an increase in echogenicity. The use of ultrasound is cost effective, non-invasive, easy and reproducible. Early detection of ultrasound abnormalities helps in reducing the progression of harmful effects.In the research carried out by Yaritza-Yelania[41], it can be seen that obesity, family history and genetic factors are risk factors that increase the possibility of suffering from renal lithiasis, due to the fact that obesity contributes to increased excretion of calcium oxalates and uric acid for their subsequent crystallisation; family history due to the epidemiological study[65], which has demonstrated its incidence and genetic factors such as: race or ethnic group, especially in countries such as Ecuador. The aforementioned studies are related to Tania González[43], who states that the main risk factors that lead to renal lithiasis are overweight, high blood pressure, hyperuricaemia and family history. Similarly, D'Achiardi et al[44] , indicate that risk factors may be non-modifiable such as age, gender, racial factors, but modifiable factors such as blood pressure, proteinuria, dyslipidemia, plasma levels of aldosterone, hyperuricaemia, alcohol and others also play a role.

CONCLUSIONS

In our study there was a predominance of patients between 60 and 69 years of age, male, white skin colour and pre-university education. Arterial hypertension was the most frequently identified pathological antecedent in the sample studied and, according to BMI, the vast majority were classified as overweight.A total of 17 patients were diagnosed in the initial stages of CKD, according to the glomerular filtration rate assessment, of which the predominant sex was male, age group 60-69 years, hypertension as the underlying disease and, according to the ultrasound assessment, the loss of the cortico-medullary relationship was identified as the most significant finding in the patients. The results of the survey showed a low level of knowledge about Chronic Kidney Disease (CKD).

RECOMMENDATIONS

Based on the main results obtained, it is necessary to establish strategies at primary health care level to reduce the incidence of this pathology.Among them, keeping blood pressure under control is essential to prevent kidney damage and it is necessary to follow a doctor's instructions to monitor blood pressure on a regular basis.For patients with diabetes, it is crucial to keep blood glucose levels within the recommended limits, as diabetes is one of the main causes of chronic kidney disease. Another important element is diet where reducing sodium intake, limiting protein intake, controlling fluid intake, increasing the amount of fruits and vegetables in the diet are key recommendations for kidney health.In relation to lifestyle, avoiding smoking and maintaining a healthy weight helps prevent diabetes, hypertension and other conditions that can lead to kidney disease. Another important element is that being physically active can help prevent obesity and improve cardiovascular health, which contributes positively to kidney health. This is why it is important to remember that prevention and treatment of chronic kidney disease should be done under the supervision of a healthcare professional. If you have associated risk factors or concerns about your kidney health, I recommend that you consult a medical specialist.

BIBLIOGRAPHICAL REFERENCES

1. Espinosa Cuevas MdA. Renal disease. Gac Med Mex [internet]. 2016 [cited 14 September 2020]; 152 Suppl 1: 90 - 96. Available from: https://www.anmm.org.mx/GMM/2016/s1/GMM_152_2016_S1_090-096.pdf

2. Sosa N, Polo RA, Méndez SN, Sosa M. Characterisation of patients with chronic kidney disease on haemodialysis. Medisur [internet]. 2016 [cited 29 Dec 2019]; 14(4): [approx. 10p.]. Available from: http://medisur.sld.cu/index.php/medisur/article/vi ew/2969\.

3. Historical background. First notes on renal diseases. Chapter 2. In: Hernando Avendaño L. Historia de la Nefrología en España. Barcelona: Ediciones Pulso; 2012. p. 19 - 20.

4. Cusumano AM, Rosa Diez G. Notes for the history of dialysis in the world and in Argentina. Second part: the beginnings of haemodialysis in Argentina. Rev Nefrol Dial Traspl [Internet]. Sep 16, 2020 [cited 2020 Nov 4]; 40(3): 242 - 250. Available from: https://www.revistarenal.org.ar/index.php/rndt/article/view/538

5. Herrera Añazco P, Pacheco Mendoza J, Taype Rondan A. Chronic kidney disease in Peru. A narrative review of published scientific articles. Acta Med Peru [internet]. 2016 [cited 2020 Nov 4]; 33(2): 130 - 137 http://www.scielo.org.pe/pdf/amp/v33n2/a07v33n2.pdf http://www.scielo.org.pe/pdf/amp/v33n2/a07v33n2.pdf.

6. Díaz Armas MT, Gómez Leyva B, Robalino Valdivieso MP, Lucero Proaño SA. Epidemiological behaviour in patients with end-stage chronic kidney disease in Ecuador. CCM [internet]. 2018 [cited 14 September 2020]; (2): 312 - 324. Available from:

http://scielo.sld.cu/pdf/ccm/v22n2/ccm11218.pdf

7. Lacomba Trejo L, Mateu Mollá J, Carbajo Álvarez E, Oltra Benavent AM, Galán Serrano A. Advanced chronic kidney disease. Association between anxiety, depression and resilience. Rev. Colomb. Nefrol [Internet]. 2019 [cited 4 September2020]; 6(2): 103 - 111. Available from: https://revistanefrologia.org/index.php/rcn/article/view/344/pdf

8. Ramírez Perdomo CA, Solano Ruíz MC. The social construction of the experience of living with chronic kidney disease. Rev. Latino-Am. Enfermagem [internet]. 2018 [cited 4 September 2020]; 26: e3028. Available from: https://www.scielo.br/pdf/rlae/v26/es_0104-1169-rlae-26-e3028.pdf; http://dx.doi.org/10.1590/1518-8345.2439.3028

9. Gorostidi M, Santamaría R, Alcázar R, Fernández Fresnedo G, Galcerán JM, Goicoechea M, et al. Spanish Society of Nephrology document on KDIGO guidelines for the evaluation and treatment of chronic kidney disease. Nefrología [internet]. 2014 [cited 14 September 2020]; 34(3): 302 - 316. Available from: http://scielo.isciii.es/pdf/nefrologia/v34n3/especial2.pdf

10. United States Renal Data System. Chapter 13: International Comparisons. In: 2015 USRDS annual data report: Epidemiology of kidney disease in the United States [Internet]. Bethesda, MD: National Institutes of Health, National Institute of Diabetes and Digestive and Kidney Diseases; 2015 [cited 16 Feb 2019]. Available from: http://www.usrds.org/2015/view/v2_13.aspx

11. Bencomo Rodríguez O. Chronic Kidney Disease: prevention is better than treatment. Rev Cubana Med Gen Integr [Internet]. 2015 [cited 5 May 2019]; 31(3): [ca.10p.].Available from: http://www.revmgi.sld.cu/index.php/mgi/article/view/66/24

12. Centro Coordinador del Programa de Atención Nacional a la Enfermedad Renal, Diálisis y Trasplante de Cuba. Cuba Nefro-Red Yearbook 2014. Situation of chronic kidney disease in Cuba 2014. 3rd year [Internet]. [cited 11 May 2019].Available at: http://files.sld.cu/nefrologia/files/2015/09/anuarionefrologia-2014-pagina-web- especialidad.pdf

13. Gonzalez Bedat MC, Rosa Diez G, Ferreiro A. The Latin American Registry of Dialysis and Renal Transplantation: the importance of the development of national registries in Latin America. Nefrología Latinoamericana [internet]. 2017 [cited 20 November 2020];14(1):12-21. Available from: https://www.elsevier.es/es- revista-nefrologia-latinoamericana-265-articulo-elregistro-latinoamericano- dialisis-trasplante-S2444903216300051

14. Fajardo Arias CR, López Salguero CS. Incidence of chronic kidney disease in patients of the Internal Medicine area of a hospital in the city of Guayaquil. [thesis]. Guayaquil, Ecuador: Universidad Católica de Santiago de Guayaquil; 2019.

15. Aldrete Velasco JA, Chiquete E, Rodríguez García JA, Rincón Pedrero R, et al. Mortality from chronic kidney disease and its relationship with diabetes in Mexico. Med Int Méx [internet]. 2018 July August [cited 14 September 2020]; 34(4):536 550.Available at: https://www.medigraphic.com/pdfs/medintmex/mim-2018/mim184d.pdf

16. Haemodialysis. National Institute of Diabetes and Digestive and Kidney Diseases. NIDDK [Internet]. 2019 [cited 2020 Jan 18]. Available from: https://www.niddk.nih.gov/health-information/informacion-delasalud/enfermedades-rinones/metodos-tratamiento-insuficiencia-renalhemodialisis.

17. World Health Organisation. Concept of quality of life in renal patients on haemodialysis. Geneva: WHO; 2016. Available in: https://www.paho.org/hq/index.php?option=com_content&view=article&id =105 42:2015-opsoms-sociedad-latinoamericana-nefrologíaenfermedad-renalmejorar-tratamiento&Itemid=1926&lang=en

18. Alarcón E. Quality of life of patients undergoing haemodialysis at the Hospital Nacional Arzobispo Loayza 2015. [Thesis]. Lima: Universidad Nacional Mayor de San Marcos; 2017.

19. Ministry of Public Health. National Directorate of Statistics. Anuario Estadístico de Salud 2017 [Internet]. Havana: MINSAP; 2018 [cited 4 May 2020]. Available at: http://files.sld.cu/bvscuba/files/2018/04/anuarioestadistico- de-salud-2017.pdf

20. Ministry of Public Health. National Directorate of Statistics. Anuario Estadístico de Salud 2019 [Internet]. Havana: MINSAP; 2020 [cited 4 May 2020]. Available from: http://files.sld.cu/bvscuba/files/2020/04/anuarioestadistico- de-salud-2019.pdf.

21. Gutiérrez Rufín M, Polanco López C. Chronic kidney disease in the elderly. Revista Finlay [internet]. 2018 [cited 2020 Mar 5]; 8(1): [ca. 7p.]. Available from: http://revfinlay.sld.cu/index.php/finlay/article/view/583

22. Medina, J. Á. R., Jiménez, K. D. Q., Munguía, J. J. S., Flores, M. L. N. Risk factors associated with chronic kidney disease in adults, observational study of a single health centre in Nicaragua: Original Article. Journal of the Ecuadorian Society of Nephrology, Dialysis and Transplantation, [Internet] (2022); 10(2), 74-81. [cited 14 June 2023] Available from: http://rev- sen.ec/index.php/revista-

nefrologia/article/view/18

23. Panduro Saavedra, N. P. Risk factors for progression in chronic kidney disease stages 1 to 3A of the hospital II Pucallpa-EsSalud 2019. (Specialty thesis). National University of Ucayali. Perú. [Internet]. (2021). [cited 11 July2023]. Available at: http://repositorio.unu.edu.pe/bitstream/handle/UNU/4732/UNU_MEDICIN A_202 1_T_NILSA-PANDURO.pdf?sequence=1&isAllowed=y

24. Moreno, Y. B., Valdés, M. A. S., López, G. C. Detection of occult chronic kidney disease in patients hospitalized in an Internal Medicine Department. Acta Médica de Cuba, [Internet] (2020). 21(1), 1-17. [cited 17 August 2023]. Available At: https://www.medigraphic.com/cgi-bin/new/resumen.cgi?IDARTICULO=97981

25 Soto Cruzado, Ó. M., Velásquez Samillán, R. F. Clinical-epidemiological characteristics of occult chronic kidney disease in patients of the older adult programme of the Carlos Castañeda Iparraguirre Essalud polyclinic 2019-2022. [Internet]. (2023). [cited 14 June 2023] Available from: https://repositorio.unprg.edu.pe/bitstream/handle/20.500.12893/11330/Sot o_Cruzado_%c3%93scar_Miguel%20y%20Vel%c3%a1squez_Samill%c3 %a1n_Ric ardo_Felipe.pdf?sequence=1&isAllowed=y

26 Sanchez Castañon, K. K. Staging of chronic renal disease in hypertensive patients from Centro at Salud 9 of Octubre-Pucallpa 2021. (Thesis speciality) Universidad Nacional de Ucayali. [Internet] (2023). [cited 11 July 2023].Available at: http://repositorio.unu.edu.pe/bitstream/handle/UNU/6040/B3_2023_UNU_ MEDI CINA_2023_T_KRISS-ANCHEZ_V1.pdf?sequence=1&isAllowed=y

27. Li, W. Y., Chiu, F. C., Zeng, J. K., Li, Y. W., Huang, S. H., Yeh, H. C.,

et al.Mobile health app with social media to support self-management for patients with chronic kidney disease: prospective randomized controlled study. Journal of medical Internet research, [Internet] (2020); 22(12), e19452 [cited 17 August 2023]. Available from: https://www.jmir.org/2020/12/e19452/

28 Okoro, R. N., Ummate, I., Ohieku, J. D., Yakubu, S. I., Adibe, M. O., Okonta, M. J. Kidney disease knowledge and its determinants among patients with chronic kidney disease. Journal of Patient Experience, [Internet] (2020); 7(6), 1303-1309. [cited 17 August 2023]. Disponible en: https://journals.sagepub.com/doi/full/10.1177/2374373520967800

29. Serra-Valdés M, Serra-Ruíz M, Viera-García M. Chronic non-communicable diseases: current magnitude and future trends. Finlay Journal. [Internet]. 2018 [cited 17 May 2018];8(2). [cited 14 June 2023] Available from: http://revfinlay.sld.cu/index.php/finlay/article/view/561

30. Barreto S, León D, Álvarez MA, Mendieta D, Oviedo L, López O, et al. Detection of occult chronic kidney disease in patients of the family health units of loma Pytaasunción. Rev. Salud Pública Parag. [journal on the internet]. 2016 [cited 11 July 2023]; 6(1). Available from: http://revistas.ins.gov.py/index. php/rspp/article /view/347/271

31 Delgado-Mejía M, Delgado-Astorga C, Ávalos-Ruvalcaba T, Paredes-Casillas P, González-González E. Control and evaluation of microalbuminuria in a population of the state of Nayarit, Mexico. Study carried out by means of self-measurement of blood pressure. Med Int Méx [online journal].2018 [cited 4 February 2020]; 34(6):864-873 Available from: https://doi.org/10. 24245/mim. v34i6.2617.

32. Rodríguez-Ramos J, Herrera-Miranda G. Risk factors related to chronic kidney disease. Policlínico Luis A. Turcios Lima, Pinar del Río,

2019. Medisur. 2022; 20(1).

33 Labrador P, González-Sanchidrián S, Polanco S, Davin E, Fuentes J, Gómez- Martino J. Detection and classification of chronic kidney disease in Primary Care and the importance of albuminuria. Semergen. [journal on the internet] 2018 [cited 4 February 2020]; 44(2): 82-89. [cited 14 June 2023] Available from:
https://doi.org/10.1016/j.semerg. 2016.11.009.
34. Kalantar-Zadeh, Li PK. Strategies to prevent kidney disease and its progression. Nat Rev Nephrol. [Internet]. 2020;16(3):129-30. [cited 11 July 2023]. Available from: https://dx.doi.org/10.1038/s41581-020-0253-1.

35. Centers for Disease Control and Prevention (CDC). Chronic Kidney Disease in the United States, 2019. Atlanta, GA: US Department of Health and Human Services, Centers for Disease Control and Prevention; 2019.

36 Chen T, Harris D. Challenges of chronic kidney disease prevention. Med J Aust. [Internet]. 2015;203(5):209-10. [cited 17 August 2023]. Available from: https://dx.doi.org/10.5694/mja15.00241.

37. HIDALGO QUIJIJE, Y. A., MOREIRA LUCAS, Y. Y. Biomarkers of kidney damage: new perspectives (Bachelor's thesis, Jipijapa-Unesum). [Internet]. (2022). [cited 17 August 2023]. Available from:
http://repositorio.unesum.edu.ec/handle/53000/4375

38. Domínguez, Y. R., Gutiérrez, H. L., Milera, A. M., Falcón, N. H., González, B.M. M. Behaviour of Chronic Kidney Disease in the elderly in Primary Care. Contreras" Polyclinic. 2017. Dominio de las Ciencias, [Internet] (2021); 7(1), 364-382. [cited 14 June 2023] Available from:
https://dialnet.unirioja.es/servlet/articulo?codigo=8385887

39. Vidal Morales, S. Y. B. Hallazgos ultrasonográficos en pacientes con sospecha y diagnóstico de enfermedad renal crónica (Doctoral dissertation,

University of San Carlos de Guatemala). [Internet]. (2020). [cited 11 July 2023]. Available from: https://core.ac.uk/download/pdf/343376963.pdf

40 Raju, N. K., Rao, J. M., Raju, D. S. S. K. Role of renal sonography in the diagnosis of chronic kidney disease. International Journal of Radiology and Diagnostic Imaging, [Internet]. (2019); 2(1), 38-41. [cited 17 August 2023]. Available In: https://web.archive.org/web/20200306232411id_/http://www.radiologypap er.co m/article/view/26/2-1-10

41 Yaritza-Yelania, Q. C., Reyes-López, A. J., Zorrilla-Cevallos, P. L. Urine crystalluria and its association with renal lithiasis in an adult population. MQRInvestigar, [Internet] (2023); 7(3), 183-202. [cited 14 June 2023] Available from: http://www.investigarmqr.com/ojs/index.php/mqr/article/view/453/1833

42. García García, P., Luis Yanes, M., García Nieto, V. Renal Lithiasis. Nefrología clínica. [Internet]. (12 2019). [cited 11 July 2023]. Available from: http://doi:10.1038/s41581-021-00513-4

43. Tania González León, M. R. Risk factors for urinary lithiasis in a population. infomed, [Internet]. (11 of 2022); III(25). [cited 17 August 2023]. Available from: https://www.bostonscientific.com/es-MX/health-conditions/calculos-renales/basics/causes-risk-factors.html.

44. Roberto D'achiardi Rey M.D, F. J. Risk factors for chronic kidney disease. Revista Med, II (19). [Internet]. (2 of 2021). [cited 14 June 2023] Available from: https://www.mayoclinic.org/es-es/diseases-conditions/chronic- kidney-disease/symptoms-causes/syc-20354521.

1- Semi-structured interview Partner:

We are conducting an investigation into chronic kidney disease. We need you to answer this inquiry as honestly as possible.

Thank you

Name and surname:

Date:

Medical History:

Age:

Sex: Male Female

Skin colour: White Black

Level of schooling

Primary Secondary

Pre-University

University

Highly educated

Weightings

Weight

Size

BMI

Personal Pathological History

Diabetes Mellitus: Obesity

HYPERTENSION Hyperlipemia Smoking Proteinuria Genetic diseases

Low birth weight Repeated urinary tract infections Other

Family Pathological History Mother

Parent

Sibling

Toxic habits

Cigarette or Tobacco Alcohol Coffee Work you do

2- Survey

a) What do you understand by a risk factor for a disease?:

b) Chronic Kidney Disease (CKD) is a disease that frequently affects the population, in which the following symptoms and signs may occur. Mark with an X the ones you think are correct

---- Urinating at night

---- Decay

---- Loss of appetite

---- Mucosa white

---- Burning when urinating

---- Frequent urination

---- Facial oedema

---- Fatigue

--- Nausea

---- Vomiting

c) Do you know any risk factors for the disease? Possible answers:

- Consumption of animal fats

- Food rich in animal and vegetable protein and grains.

- Arterial hypertension

- Diabetes mellitus

- Excessive salt consumption

- Smoking

- Urinary tract obstruction

d) If you or your family member has any symptoms of Chronic Kidney Disease, what should you do?
Taking tablets that have been prescribed by your doctor for other conditions.illnesses.

-See your nearest doctor as a matter of urgency.

-Frequent checking of glycaemia and blood pressure.

Take recommended home remedies for them.

Take measures to prevent other family members from getting sick.
e) As a person at risk, you consider that you could ever develop chronic kidney disease.
f) Do you consider CKD to be a threat to your health?
Yes No Why?
g) What measures do you consider necessary to prevent Chronic Kidney Disease.
Possible answers

Consumption of low-salt diets

Practising physical exercise

Controlling blood pressure.

Avoid repeated urinary tract infections.

-Consistent consumption of fruit and vegetables

-Eliminate consumption of foods rich in animal fats.

Avoid a sedentary lifestyle and smoking.

Avoiding high blood sugar levels

h) Are you adhering to your treatment for your chronic non-communicable disease?

i) Know the main complications of chronic kidney disease. Name some of them.

3. Questionnaire to specialists.

Dear Specialist:

You have been selected for your knowledge and experience to be part of a group of specialists who will evaluate the proposal of Community Intervention for the early diagnosis of Chronic Kidney Disease in the population at risk belonging to CMF 19-47 belonging to Policlínico Capitán Roberto Fleites.

General data:

Name and surname:

Teaching category:

Speciality:

Years of experience   :

Express your considerations about the system of educational actions in terms of:

• Relevance: Whether the way it is designed responds to the difficulties identified in the diagnosis.

• Feasibility: Real possibility of availability of human and material resources to actually implement the system of educational actions.

• Structure: Whether or not it conforms to what is established for a system of educational actions.

• Utility: Whether the product designed responds to older adults' lack of knowledge about medicine use.

• Scientific-pedagogical value: If the results obtained obey a good harmony between organisation, methodology, appropriate language and up-to-date research carried out through a rigorous research process.

The evaluative categories should be given a value from 5 to 1.

Aspects to evaluate	1	2	3	4	5
Relevance					
Feasibility					
Structure					
Utility					
Scientific-pedagogical value					

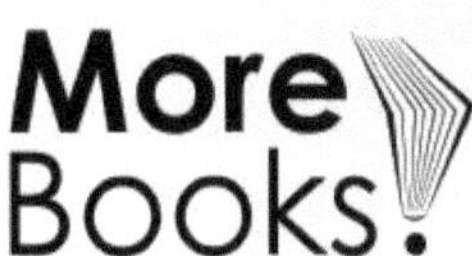

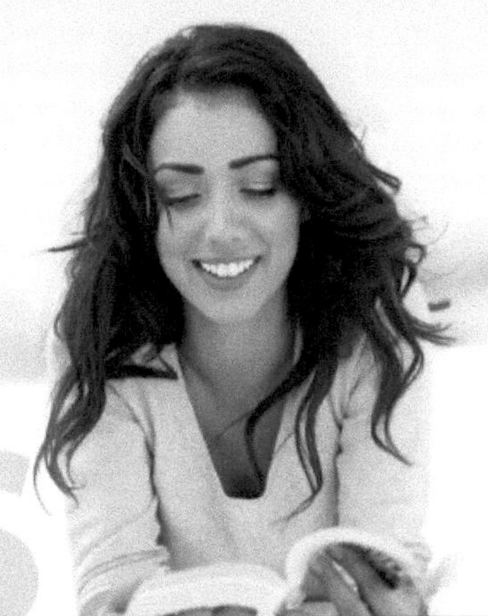

Buy your books fast and straightforward online - at one of world's fastest growing online book stores! Environmentally sound due to Print-on-Demand technologies.

Buy your books online at
www.morebooks.shop

Kaufen Sie Ihre Bücher schnell und unkompliziert online – auf einer der am schnellsten wachsenden Buchhandelsplattformen weltweit! Dank Print-On-Demand umwelt- und ressourcenschonend produziert.

Bücher schneller online kaufen
www.morebooks.shop

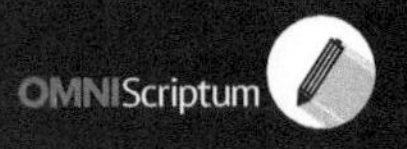

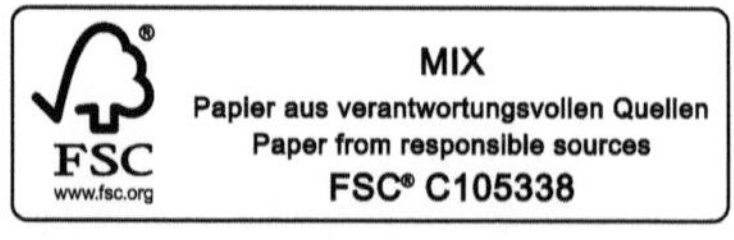

Printed by Books on Demand GmbH, Norderstedt / Germany